Alkaline Teas

Wake Up Slimmer, Feel More Energized
and Reduce Stress with Delicious Herbal
Infusions and Healing Tea Recipes

By Marta "Wellness" Tuchowska

Copyright ©Marta Tuchowska 2018

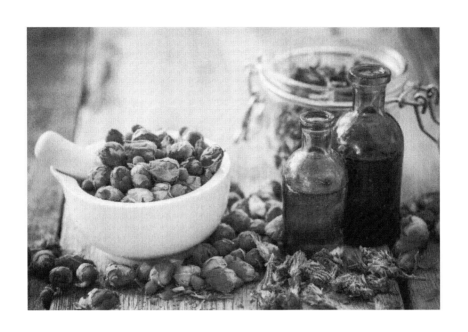

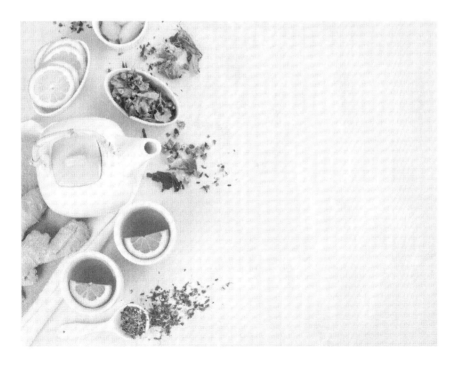

Contents

Part 1: Introduction to Alkaline Teas

Do you want to feel more energized in a natural, sustainable way?

How about getting rid of toxins and turning your body into a real health machine?

Would you like to experience unlimited mental focus and clarity while giving your body a myriad of nutrients so that it can function for you at its optimal levels?

Perhaps you have been eating healthily but are still looking for that next level and wondering what to do to optimize your healthy lifestyle.

Maybe you are just starting out but have already made up your mind. You already know what you want.

You want to transform, and you simply need someone to guide you in the right direction so that you can take powerful action that aligns with your vision. The new you. Energized. Glowing. Healthy. Peaceful. And a huge inspiration to those around you.

If that's you, you have picked the right book and I am here to congratulate you on making that investment.

It's more than a book on how to stay hydrated. It's a book that will help you revolutionize your lifestyle and experience new levels of wellness and clarity as well as physical and emotional fitness.

You see, it's not only about what you eat. It's also about how you live and what you drink.

Most people sabotage their healthy diets with poor hydration, or no hydration at all. What they choose to drink is not helpful at all and it poisons their body while making their mind less alert.

Many people just run on caffeine. And it's not a big secret- too much caffeine makes us anxious, dehydrated and prone to stress. In fact, I always say that drinking too much caffeine is like drinking stress hormones and asking for trouble.

Not a very pleasant place to be.

That is why I am writing this book. I want to introduce you to alkaline teas and infusions that will help you reduce your caffeine intake and feel energized naturally, as you deserve to.

Not only that, but you will quickly learn how you can use alkaline tea recipes to help you reduce, or get rid of, many common ailments like headaches, insomnia, poor digestion, low energy levels, lack of focus, sugar cravings, colds, and flu.

The recipes in this book can be used as warm drinks- this is what they are known for anyway. It feels so good to treat yourself to a nice, warm relaxing tea or infusion and there is always an excuse to do so, right?

Most teas can also be served cooled down, with ice cubes and infused with fruit.

When you dive into the recipes, you will see how much creativity is involved.

Whenever creating recipes for you, I like to present them in such a way that you understand how many different options there are.

My intention is to always make sure you find at least a few recipes you will enjoy and stick to for the long term to get the wellness benefits that you want.

At the same time, I like to create recipes that help stimulate your imagination and motivation so that you feel empowered to create your own recipes, based on your own experiments.

Now, back to our teas. Alkaline teas.

You may be wondering why they are called "alkaline".

At the end of this chapter there will be a brief summary of the alkaline diet, so in case you are new to it, please don't worry.

However, for the time being, we will keep it very, very uncomplicated so that you get hooked on the world of healing, caffeine-free infusions even before we get into the recipes and all the explanations.

The reason that the recipes in this book are called "alkaline" is simple. They form a part of the Alkaline Diet and Lifestyle army.

You see, the alkaline diet focuses on feeding your body with foods (and drinks) that are packed with nutrients and are easy to digest. That is really the simplest explanation there is.

At the same time, when it comes to drinks, it focuses on pure hydration- that is, drinks that contain no sugar and no caffeine.

This is something that most people overlook. First of all, because of a lack of information and secondly, because coffee and caffeine drinks are very popular and are also addictive.

Before we dive any deeper, I want to make a few things clear.

#1 There is nothing wrong about enjoying coffee and caffeine drinks every now and then. It's absolutely fine. However, the problem is when we are depending on them and can't even focus properly without overindulging in huge amounts of caffeine.

#2 I am very open-minded when it comes to different diets and nutritional lifestyles and I absolutely hate preaching to people.

Not my thing at all.

Also, most of the unhealthy habits that I point out as habits to avoid are the same poor habits I was guilty of in the past before I decided to transform. Very often it's like me giving advice to the younger me from the past.

It is my hope that you will benefit from what I am sharing here, and that the way I share it will make you feel empowered and motivated to take meaningful action so that you can achieve your health goals in an easy, fun and exciting way.

The last thing I want to do is to preach.

Now, back to coffee and caffeine addiction. I will open up a bit and tell you where I was a few years ago. Maybe you can relate.

I had basically reached a stage where my addiction to coffee was so strong that I could not think nor operate without it.

As with all addictions, I needed more and more of it. I would sit in my office and stare at my computer, experiencing a big headache. That would make me think that I needed another coffee. Because of that, I was feeling overstimulated and nervous. I could not sleep well.

I would wake up at night feeling anxious. At the same time, I knew I was damaging my health. I was already on the healthy eating path and was learning about the alkaline diet. I knew that too much caffeine was a big no-no.

Finally, I reached a point where I knew I had to shift to a caffeine-free lifestyle or at least reduce caffeine.

That decision literally changed my life. I discovered so many amazing teas and herbal infusions to experiment with.

I also created a very simple process that allowed me to gradually reduce my caffeine intake and create a stronger and more energized version of myself.

Thanks to that one simple decision, I was able to help not only myself but I was also able to inspire thousands of people around the world thanks to my books such as *Alkaline Juicing, Alkaline Smoothies, Alkaline Drinks, How to Lose Massive Weight with the Alkaline Diet, Mindfulness for Busy People* and also thanks to my recent online course the *Alkaline Diet Lifestyle* as well as my website *Holistic Wellness Project*.

This book is a natural extension of my work and it's coming to fruition because of many requests I was getting from my readers and clients.

For example, I know people who are not that much into smoothies and are looking for alkaline tea recipes which they find easier to begin with. In many cases, people are looking for something they can also use at work, and it's much easier to use your break to make a quick tea rather than make a smoothie or a juice.

Ideally, you want to add all the alkaline hydration elements- alkaline teas, smoothies, and juices. At the end of this book, there is a little bonus with the best of my alkaline green smoothie recipes for you to enjoy. Many of these recipes can be used as a meal replacement.

Honestly, I think you need all the alkaline hydration options, so to optimize your results, I suggest that aside from teas, you also focus on juices and smoothies.

However, as the title suggests, this book is 100% about tea recipes. If you want to learn more about alkaline juicing and alkaline smoothies then I recommend you check out the books I have written on that topic (you will find them at: www.holisticwellnessproject.com/books).

That being said, or rather written, congratulations on picking up this book.

Not only will you learn something new, but you will also feel inspired to make a lasting change in your life and add more variety to your diet. A diet is not only about what you eat but also about what you drink. Yes, I am repeating that time and time again.

One of my early mistakes with the alkaline diet was that I didn't know much about hydration. I thought I was doing well as I was drinking some water here and there. However, the amounts of caffeine I was consuming were actually spoiling all my alkaline diet efforts.

After I drastically changed my lifestyle by focusing on alkaline drinks and my hydration- here I refer to drinks that are sugar-free, caffeine-free and super rich in natural vitamins and minerals, I was able to create the transformation I wanted.

This is exactly what I am teaching through my online course the *AlkalineDietLifestyle.com* and this particular book.

After releasing dozens of guides on the alkaline diet and also helping people through my recipes, tips, and programs, I began to notice certain patterns.

For example, a lot of people were asking me this question:

"Marta, I don't get it. It looks like I am eating pretty much alkaline, but I am still not feeling energized. Am I doing something wrong?"

My answer usually contains the following questions:

-What do you mean by eating pretty much alkaline? (adding a little salad once a week doesn't really cut it. It's hard to see the benefits, while you don't need to be perfect, about 70% of your diet should be fresh, alkaline, plant-based unprocessed foods. More on that later).

-What do you drink? What about your hydration?

In most cases, the culprits are poor hydration or drinks that are not at all alkaline forming (because of high levels of sugar, especially processed sugar and caffeine).

However, after embracing a balanced, clean food diet that encompasses lots of plant-based and alkaline foods (again it's all about balance, it's not about eating 100% alkaline) and also adding lots of caffeine-free infusions and alkaline juices, a person is able to experience the miraculous benefits of the alkaline diet lifestyle. When I say *miraculous*, I refer to this amazing feeling of holistic wellness. Just feeling good, looking good and connecting with the divine part of you.

Perhaps you already know what the alkaline diet is. If that is the case, you can jump straight to the recipes now.

However, if you are new to the alkaline diet concepts, this short summary will help you quickly understand what it's all about.

This book, as the title suggests, is only about the alkaline tea recipes. However, to dive deeper, I highly recommend that you explore my other books from the series.

The alkaline diet is not a diet but a lifestyle. It encourages you to add more alkalizing foods and drinks to your diet so that your body can heal itself naturally. How?

Alkaline Diet Crash Course - Understand the Basics

According to the National Institute of Health, the pH of most of our crucial cellular and other body fluids like blood is designed to be at a pH of 7.4 which is slightly alkaline.

(you will also find resources pointing to 7.365, which is very close to 7.4).

The body has an intricate system in place to maintain that healthy, slightly alkaline pH level no matter what you eat. This is an argument that many alkaline diet skeptics use, and I get it. It's 100% true, and I say the same thing.

This is not the goal of the alkaline diet. We just can't make our blood's pH more alkaline or "higher." Our body tries to work hard for us to help maintain our ideal pH.We can't have a pH of 8 or 9. If we did, we would be dead. It's not about magically raising your pH.

The focus of the alkaline diet is to give your body the nourishment and healing tools that it needs to MAINTAIN that optimal pH almost effortlessly.

If we fail to do so, we torture our body with incredible stress! Yes, when the body has to continually work overtime to detoxify all of the cells and maintain our pH, it finally succumbs to disease.

Let me name a few examples of what can happen if we continuously eat an acid-forming diet (also called SAD - Standard American Diet) and drink too much caffeine and sugar that does not support our body at all. Our body ends up sick and tired of working overtime and may manifest one or more of the following conditions:

- Constant inflammation

- Immune and hormonal imbalance

- Lack of energy, mental fog- and you go for another cup of coffee yet still feel the same

- Yeast and candida overgrowth

- Digestive damage

- Weakened bones. Our body is forced to pull minerals like magnesium and calcium from our bones to maintain the alkaline balance it needs for constant healing processes.

In summary, eating more alkaline foods, for example veggies, herbs, and greens, helps support our body so that it can work for us at optimal levels while eating more acidic food (aka processed food, fast food etc.) doesn't help at all. The alkaline diet is not about magically raising our pH, but helping our body rebalance itself by supporting its natural healing functions.

Why is it called an alkaline diet, then?

To be honest, I don't know. It could also be called the Eat More Veggies diet, or perhaps Veggie Lover Diet, but then most people would never even look at it. I guess that it was called the alkaline diet for a reason, probably to make it more mysterious and sexy so that there is this "hook" that makes people think, "Hmmm, what is it? That stuff must be hot!"

The alkaline diet is sisters with a clean food diet, anti-inflammatory diet, vegetarian diet, vegan diet, macrobiotic diet, and the raw food diet. In fact, it offers an incredible blend and the best of them all. All of those diets that are more in the plant-based diet category.

However, it's not only about what we eat. It's also about how we live and what we think. It's not just a diet; it's a lifestyle. If you want vibrant health and alkaline wellness, try to go outdoors more. Meditate, laugh, spend time with family and friends, do things you enjoy so that you can de-stress, and practice mindfulness. It's not only about nutrition. It's about your lifestyle. Again, this is exactly the message I share on my social media, my website and through my books.

A huge part of that lifestyle is what we drink.

I warmly encourage you to use this book to your advantage. Set a simple, process-oriented goal to begin with. This strategy is what's proven to work for most people and personally I love focusing on process-oriented goals (while of course, making sure those goals align with my long-term health and wellness vision- for me it's constant transformation and taking others on that incredible journey too so that we can all empower and energize the planet!).

A process-oriented goal is for example when you decide to swap your afternoon coffee for a caffeine-free infusion. Or, create a morning or evening ritual where you enjoy a nice cup of alkaline tea, meditate, read or do something you enjoy. Just to spend some time with yourself and give yourself a well-deserved moment of reflection and meditation.

Whatever works for you, be my guest!

To learn more about the alkaline diet & lifestyle (the practical way, so that you can start transforming your body and mind), be sure to sign up for my free Alkaline Wellness Newsletter at:

www.HolisticWellnessProject.com/alkaline

When you join you will receive free instant access to these alkaline cuties (I only share them with my VIP subscribers):

3 Free Bonus Guides

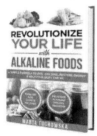
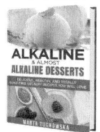
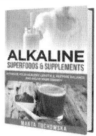

+more valuable tips, recipes and inspiration delivered to your inbox.

PART 2 Alkaline Tea Recipes

So why is a caffeine-free lifestyle or low caffeine (probably easier for most people out there) lifestyle good for you?

Let's have a look at some facts about what overdoing caffeine can do to your health.

What too much caffeine does to you:

-First of all, you experience anxiety and insomnia because of getting overstimulated with caffeine. As I explained earlier in the intro of this book it is a vicious cycle...

I have been there as well and it's not the best place to be at, to be honest, because no matter what you do you can't relax and unwind. Your mind is always over-active, you think about your to-do list and just feel sorry for yourself.

Yes, caffeine in small amounts is fine and it can help us stay alert. Many people use it as motivation to be up early, but it also blocks the sleep-inducing chemicals in the brain while stimulating adrenaline production.

So, if you want to enjoy a better sleep, I would highly recommend that you get rid of caffeine in the afternoons.

-Headaches- these are basically caffeine withdrawal symptoms.

Some people are more prone to them than others. For many people, it is an invitation to enjoy another cup of coffee or any caffeinated drink.

However, what I would recommend instead are a nice herbal infusion and a gentle head and face self-massage.

You can use any natural cream or oil, such as for example coconut oil and add a couple of drops of lavender or mint essential oil. Chamomile and fennel essential oils are great too. Massage your forehead and temples, making sure to avoid the eye area. You can also massage your neck and scalp.

That will help you relieve a headache and break the vicious cycle so that you can start reducing your caffeine intake.

Another interesting thing is that some people never develop a strong caffeine addiction. They just have a mini coffee habit, like for example drinking one quality expresso early in the morning.

They never feel tempted to drink more of it. Nor do they suffer from any withdrawal symptoms if they skip their coffee rituals.

Unfortunately, some people do develop caffeine addiction, whether they want to admit it or not.

Another sign of overdoing coffee and caffeine, in general, are stomach aches...

-Stomach aches- combined with the previous side effects are a bad trio!

Perhaps you have experienced that feeling of discomfort after drinking a cup of coffee or even black tea. You were hoping to get more alert, however, the stomach pain got so strong, you could not concentrate, and you just wanted for it to go away. I have been there and I can tell you this- it's a very scary place to be. You just don't feel productive.

You would probably feel a huge sense of relief after drinking a nice herbal infusion like fennel tea. Alternatively, some clean, filtered water infused with some herbs.

At the same time, overdoing coffee and caffeine inhibits iron absorption and depletes your body of vital alkaline minerals such as magnesium. Not the best place to be.

The unpleasant combination of all the side effects listed above also leads to another issue.

You may end up craving something sweet. More sugar, more acidity, and the vicious cycle continues.

As one of my health mentors, Yuri Elkaim says, "You crave what's in your blood".

That is why it's important to break that vicious cycle starting right here right now.

Oh, Marta, what am I getting into? Does that mean I will never be able to enjoy your cup of coffee?

Of course not.

Balance is the key and it's created by creating progress in all areas of your health.

With a healthy, balanced, clean-food diet in place you will already be on the right track. This means a diet that includes lots of fresh, unprocessed alkaline foods, veggies, and salads, plus optimal hydration and relaxation, you will already be living a healthy, balanced lifestyle.

So, it's absolutely fine to enjoy one cup of coffee a day if you really need to. Make sure it's quality, organic coffee though. You could also experiment with some green tea, which can actually be helpful while transitioning to a caffeine-free or low caffeine lifestyle (green tea is not caffeine-free though).

How to transition to a caffeine-free or caffeine low lifestyle when you have headaches etc.?

The tips below will help you make this transition painlessly.

Tip # 1 Dilute your coffee with coconut or almond milk (these are considered alkaline-forming plant-based kinds of milk). You could even make a healthy plant-based latte or cappuccino. Then, gradually increase the amount of milk while adding less and less coffee. You can also add a teaspoon of coconut oil. It's like a famous bulletproof coffee but with plant-based, dairy-free milk in it.

You can still enjoy the taste and smell of coffee in the morning, and you will notice that it's very often the smell that helps you wake up and you can do with less and less caffeine. It's a really liberating feeling.

Tip# 2 Start your day with a glass of warm water with some lemon. That will really wake you up. Very often we feel tired and grumpy as we are actually dehydrated. By focusing on hydration and adding some lemon to it (lemons are alkaline forming fruits because they are low in sugar and high in alkaline-forming minerals such as magnesium and calcium) you will feel more energized.

Tip# 3 Tea is less aggressive than coffee. Green and black tea are not completely caffeine free, but you can make some black tea with coconut milk or rice milk. Just don't make it too strong.

You can also try some green tea with fennel tea and grapefruit juice. If you can't stand grapefruit juice (many people can't, I know I know, I am a bit of a weirdo and a grapefruit juice addict), then, simply stick to a mixture of green tea and fennel tea. Wow, amazing!

Green tea also blends well with mint. It's actually the famous Moroccan tea recipe. (Just don't add tons of sugar like the original recipe encourages you to do. You can do very well without it or add some stevia).

Of course, focus on experimenting with the recipes from this book that are caffeine free.

From my own experience, I know that the side effects of quitting coffee are not the best place to be. Headaches, lack of focus, irritability. I remember when I first went through a caffeine-free regime…that was a few years ago…oh boy, did I feel irritated! And in pain…

Going cold turkey works for sure, but you must be very strong-willed.

Another way is to do it gradually so that your body doesn't react to your caffeine-free lifestyle change by torturing you with the headaches aka the withdrawal symptoms.

That is why most people go for a balanced solution and get rid of their coffee addiction step by step.

Again, as I said, your goal can be a caffeine free lifestyle or an almost caffeine-free lifestyle. Both are fine. It's not about being perfect.

I drink lots of herbal teas and live an alkaline lifestyle, but every now and then I also enjoy some coffee and green tea and doing very well. Balance and progress always win over perfection.

So now, some technicalities...how do I make my tea?

There are 2 ways to go about it:

You can use teabags, and this is much easier, especially if you want to take your teas with you. You can also easily mix different teabags.

Or you can get the tea in seeds or powder and use a teapot, or a tea infuser.

There are many of them available online. Simply search for tea mug, tea mug with infuser etc.

The best way to use this book for optimal benefits:

You need to make sure you eat a healthy, clean food diet and avoid processed foods.

I also recommend that you try to explore more plant-based options (even if you are not fully vegan) and gluten-free options (even if you're not celiac).

1)Eliminate processed foods from your diet and say "no" to colas and sodas - There are copious additives and preservatives in these foods. They have been known to create hormone imbalances, make you tired, and add to acidity to your body. It's just not natural for humans to consume those conveniently processed foods. The label may even say "low in calories" or "low in fat," but it will not help you in your long-term weight loss or health efforts. To start losing weight naturally, your body needs foods that are jam-packed with nutrients. Real, living foods. This, in turn, will help your body maintain its optimal blood pH (7.35) almost effortlessly.

2)Add more raw foods to your diet - especially lots of vegetables and leafy greens as well as fruits that are naturally low in sugar. Limes, lemons, grapefruits, avocados, tomatoes, and pomegranates are alkaline-forming fruits.

3)Reduce or eliminate animal products – These are extremely acid-forming. The good news is that there are many plant-based options out there and many ways to create delicious alkaline-friendly and plant-based meals that you will love! If I can do it, you can do it too.

(In case you're a meat eater, be sure to add a ton of veggies too. Same with fish or eggs, only go for local and organic and serve with a bunch of veggies).

But, honestly- plant based options are so abundant and it's easy to create tasty recipes with no animal products.

I highly recommend you check my other recipe books, like *Alkaline Salads* or *Plant Based Cookbook*).

4)Drink plenty of clean, filtered water, preferably alkaline water or fruit-infused water. Of course, also drink herbal infusions which is what this book is all about.

5)Add more vegetable juices to your diet — these are a great way to give your body more nutrients and alkalinity that will result in more energy, less inflammation, and if desired, natural weight loss.

Vegetable juices are the best shots of health! I have also written a book called *Alkaline Juicing* if you want to give it a try and want to juice the right way. If you don't like veggies, you can start juicing them and get all those condensed nutrients in almost effortlessly.

6)Reduce or eliminate processed grains, "crappy carbs," and yeast - Again, these are very acid-forming. Personally, I recommend quinoa instead (naturally gluten-free), amaranth (super nutritious), brown rice, or soba noodles (made from buckwheat and naturally gluten-free).

You can also use gluten-free wraps or make your own bread. Fruit is also an excellent natural source of carbohydrates and is great for energy. Plus, fruit always makes a great snack. Even if you are not a celiac, I highly recommend you start reducing gluten. You will feel much more alert, lighter and more focused.

Your Wellness Goals- How Do You Want to Feel?

Be specific. If you are new to setting goals, it may seem very weird at first. You may be thinking: "Who am I to be deciding on what I want to happen?" Well, that is where I can help you. You need empowerment. Right here, right now.

You can no longer be floating around just hoping something might happen. You want to make it happen and enjoy the process.

I can tell you this- the moment you decide to transform, the rest is easy.

So here's a little homework:

Write it down:

I /YOUR NAME/ deserve to be feeling amazing and enjoy unstoppable energy.

I feel worthy and deserving of /ADD YOUR GOAL HERE/

It's also important how you word the goal. If you say, "I want to lose weight", I would recommend that you rather say, "wake up slimmer", "feel lighter", or even "feel aligned with my ultimate vision". Some people say it's woo-woo. Maybe it is, but it works. I do it all the time to make sure I stay on track and reach new levels of transformation while helping other people transform too.

Your self-image is very important.

I always encourage my dear readers and clients to take action from a place of abundance and confidence, and not from a place of fear, scarcity and "trying" while not even feeling worthy of deep change and holistic transformation.

I am here to tell you that you are an amazing human being capable of much more you think you are capable of.

Value your health and wellbeing. Take care of your energy. Be patient and keep going. You will be positively surprised by the results. Your transformation and unstoppable energy.

That is real self-love. Loving yourself right here right now and taking action from that beautiful place. The place where you are already good enough, super healthy and strong.

If you're having a bad day or feeling like you are getting off track remember that Marta loves you.

Now, we can finally try the recipes!

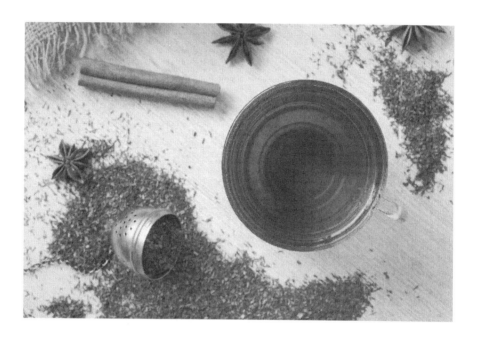

Disclaimer:

This is a simple to follow recipe and lifestyle book to inspire and motivate you on your wellness quest. However, it is not meant to diagnose or treat any medical conditions.

If you are suffering from any chronic disease, have recently undergone any medical treatment, are pregnant, lactating or suffering from any serious health condition, you need to see your doctor first.

It is also recommended that you familiarize yourself with all the precautions that the extended use of certain herbs entails. Some herbs may interfere with certain medications, and so if you take any, be sure to seek a professional advice first.

All information in this book has been carefully researched and checked for factual accuracy. However, the author and publishers make no warranty, expressed or implied, that the information contained herein is appropriate for every individual, situation or purpose, and assume no responsibility for errors or omission. The reader assumes the risk and full responsibility for all actions and the author will not be held liable for any loss or damage, whether consequential, incidental, and special or otherwise, that may result from the information presented in this publication.

Part 3 Alkaline Teas and Infusions

Recipe Measurements Used in the Recipes

The cup measurement I use is the American Cup measurement.

I also use it for dry ingredients. If you are new to it, let me help you:

If you don't have American Cup measures, just use a metric or imperial liquid measuring jug and fill your jug with your ingredient to the corresponding level. Here's how to go about it:

1 American Cup= 250ml= 8 fl.oz

For example:

If a recipe calls for 1 cup of almonds, simply place your almonds into your measuring jug until it reaches the 250 ml/8oz mark.

Quite easy, right?

I hope you found it helpful. I know that different countries use different measurements and I wanted to make things simple for you. I have also noticed that very often those who are used to American Cup measurements complain about metric measurements and vice versa. However, if you apply what I have just explained, you will find it easy to use both.

Now, let's get into recipes, that's why we are here, right?

Recipe Preparation

Most of the recipes I create and share are designed for busy people who are looking for fast solutions. With every new book, I want to make it even simpler and faster.

In alignment with that, there is no complicated preparation involved (although I'll admit, I have been guilty of that in some of my earlier books).

The tools I recommend you get, that by the way, if you are a tea person, I bet you already have, are a teacup with an infuser. We actually have quite a few of those around the house.

Then, you can also use a simple teapot, also with an infuser or a sieve, that will allow you to get rid of the infused herbs so that you can enjoy the pure tea. Although, to be honest, sometimes I like to leave out herbs like fennel or mint.

However, by doing that, I am prone to getting lots of herbs stuck between my teeth which can be annoying. So, in most cases, I use the sieve.

Precautions

I have already mentioned that the recipes in this book are not designed for self-medication or the treatment of any chronic diseases.

They are simple wellness and self-care recipes that form a part of a healthy, balanced lifestyle, in addition to a balanced diet. The teas are not to be used as meal replacements or any weird detoxes.

Any serious medical conditions must be discussed with your doctor.

Water to Use in the Recipes

I highly recommend that you use clean, filtered water.

Avoid tap water, as, in most cases and in most areas, it will be full of toxins.

You don't need any advanced equipment to get started.

However, I recommend that you get a simple water pitcher with a filter. These can be easily found online.

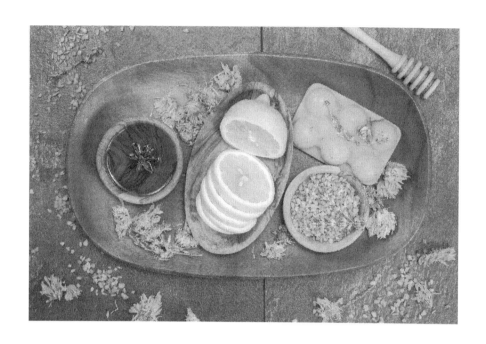

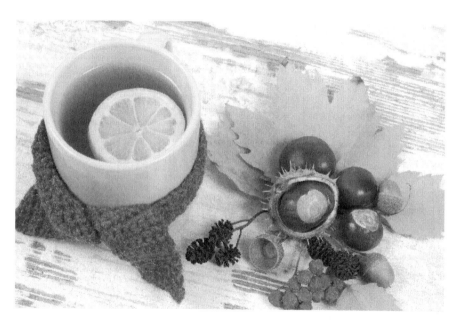

Recipe # 1 Pepper Mint Chamomile Tea with a Twist

This recipe is just a classic relaxing, caffeine-free infusion and something to really look forward to, especially after a busy day. Now, it's time to relax!

Serves: 1- 2

Ingredients:

- 1 cup boiling water
- 1 teaspoon mint leaves or mint tea
- 1 teaspoon chamomile tea
- 1 teaspoon parsley leaves, washed
- a few dates, pitted
- ½ cup coconut milk
- 1 teaspoon coconut oil
- ½ teaspoon cinnamon
- Optional: ½ teaspoon ashwagandha powder

Instructions:

1. Using a teapot or a tea mug, combine mint, chamomile, and parsley with boiling water.
2. Let infuse for approx. 10 minutes.
3. In the meantime, blend coconut milk with a few dates. Add cinnamon and coconut milk and blend again. You can easily use a small hand blender for this step.
4. This step is optional- you can slightly heat up the coconut milk.
5. Now, finalize your tea, by separating the leaves from the infusion.

6. Place the infusion in a cup and add the cinnamon-date coconut milk. So yummy! (It even stands as a separate recipe).
7. You can also add some ashwagandha powder for its relaxing and rebalancing properties. Enjoy and relax. This recipe is so soothing!

Recipe #2 Lavender and Mint Anti-Stress Tea

This is a very simple herbal recipe that I love to use with my evening meditation. It's thanks to this recipe that I manage to stick to this habit.

It's always good to have something healthy to look forward to.

Serves: 2-3

Ingredients:

•1 teaspoon lavender flowers (you can also use Melissa or verbena instead)

•2 teaspoons mint leaves, washed

•1 cup of filtered, boiling water

Instructions:

1. Using a tea mug or a pot with an infuser, combine boiling water with lavender and mint.
2. Allow to infuse for 5-10 minutes.
3. Strain and serve.
4. You can also sweeten it with some stevia if you choose to.

Lavender has various properties in terms of protecting mental health. It is used to help chase away depression and also helps in bringing about mental peace. I call it holistic wellness self-care!

Recipe #3 Almond Milk and Rosemary Tea

Since many beginners may have a hard time with ingredients like rosemary offered as a pure infusion, this recipe is just perfect because it uses other ingredients as well, therefore creating a nice, warm and tasty experience.

Rosemary is very helpful in fighting colds, flu and strengthening your immune system too.

Serves: 1-2

Ingredients:

•1 cup almond milk (or coconut milk or rice milk)

•2 tablespoons rosemary tea

•1/4 cup water, filtered, boiling

•a few dates, pitted

Instructions:

1. In a cup, combine the rosemary and the boiling water. Add the dates and cover to infuse for about 10 mins.
2. In the meantime, warm up the almond milk.
3. Strain the tea. You can leave the dates if you want.
4. Now, combine the tea with the milk.
5. Stir well and enjoy!

Recipe #4 Ayurvedic Alkaline Healing Tea

This tea is one of my favorites for meditation.

It's also very soothing, and because of the combination of ingredients it offers, it is very high in anti-inflammatory properties.

Don't worry if you don't have all the ingredients. The recipe will still be soothing and abundant even if you skip one of the ingredients.

Serves: 1-2

Ingredients:

- 1 lemon, juiced
- 4 teaspoons ginger, finely chopped
- 2 garlic cloves, peeled
- 2 tablespoons cardamom
- 1 tablespoon clove
- 1 tablespoon mint leaves, washed
- 2 cups of water, filtered, boiling

Instructions:

1. In a teapot or cup, combine the ginger, garlic, cardamom and clove and boiling water. Set aside to infuse for 10 minutes.
2. When ready, cool down a bit, by adding a bit of cold water and then add lemon juice.

(When adding lemon juice, you don't want to be adding it into boiling water or boiling tea, that is why it's better to wait until your tea is cool enough to drink it but at the same time still nice and warm).

3. Garnish with mint leaves and enjoy!

Recipe #5 Simple Healing Creamy Infusion

This is a very simple combination of various healing ingredients to help you unwind.

I especially recommend it in the winter to help you fight colds and flu.

Serves: 2

Ingredients:

- 2 cups coconut milk (you can also use almond milk, or any other plant-based milk of your choice)
- 2 cloves garlic, peeled
- 1/2 cup parsley, washed
- 1/2 cup mint, washed
- 4 inches ginger, cut in smaller pieces
- 1 teaspoon coconut oil

Instructions:

1. Place the coconut milk in a small pot and put it to boil, using low heat.
2. Add garlic, parsley, mint, and ginger.
3. Stir well and cover.
4. Switch off the heat when boiling.
5. Keep everything in a pot, covered for about 5-10 minutes for it to infuse better.
6. Then, using a sieve, strain the infusion and pour the milk into a cup.
7. Add 1 teaspoon of coconut oil and enjoy!

Recipe #6 Simple Rosehip Tea with a Twist

If you are a fan of all in one solutions, this is the recipe for you.

Rosehip tea is your holistic tool to help you have healthy, beautiful skin, fight colds, detoxify your body and strengthen your immune system.

It's also great to prevent inflammation and prevent cardiovascular diseases. You can enjoy this recipe as it is- warm, in the winter, or you could turn it into a super-healthy iced tea to enjoy in the summer.

Serves: 1-2

Ingredients:

- 1 teaspoon rosehip tea
- 1 cup water, filtered, boiling
- 2 dates, pitted
- 2 inches of ginger
- 2 slices of lemon
- 1 cinnamon stick

Instructions:

1. In a teapot or cup, combine the boiling water with rosehip tea, dates, and ginger.
2. Let infuse for about 10-mins.
3. Now, strain and serve with 2 slices of lemon with 1 cinnamon stick.
4. Enjoy!

Suggestions:

1. You can also sweeten it with stevia or maple syrup.
2. If you are looking to add more detox properties, I would recommend you mix the tea with some freshly squeezed grapefruit juice. In that case, first make sure your tea is slightly cooled down (to where you can drink it) before adding the grapefruit juice

Recipe #7 Caffeine Addicts' Infusion

Please note, this recipe is an exception as it does contain caffeine.

Treat it as a bonus recipe, one of those recipes to help you transition away from drinking too much coffee.

I used to be a coffee person and quitting caffeine was a big challenge for me. While yerba mate is not 100% alkaline (it contains caffeine, and caffeine is not considered alkaline), it is full of antioxidants. It also helps stimulate weight loss. I use yerba mate as well as green tea occasionally. If you are a coffee addict wanting to kick your habit, you might notice headaches. Therefore I suggest you use green tea or yerba mate to help you transition. Mix it with other herbs to balance it (herbs are alkaline).

Ever since a friend of mine, originally from Argentina, introduced me to yerba mate, I fell in love with it!

Also, traditionally, mate is drunk from *bombilla*, which in Argentinian Spanish is pronounced as *bombisha*. There is a whole ritual around it, which I am sure could be a book in itself. However, for the purpose of this book, we will keep it very simple.

Yerba mate can be also found in teabags, and although I am pretty sure it is not an ideal solution for most Argentinians, who like using their *bombishas*. I it's totally OK on a busy day or for a yerba mate noobie.

Serves: 2-3

Ingredients:

•2 tablespoons yerba mate, or 2 mate teabags

•2-3 cups filtered water, warm but not boiling

•2 tablespoons mint

Instructions:

1. Place the water in a pot and allow it to simmer.
2. Make sure that it does not boil.
3. Place the yerba mate in a glass.
4. Add in the mint leaves and mix.
5. Add the 5 tablespoons of warm water to it and allow the leaves to rise up. Wait a few minutes.
6. Keep the temperature of the water around 170°F (75°C).
7. Now, pour the rest of the water into the glass and allow it to stand for a few minutes.
8. Pour the tea through a strainer and serve warm.
9. Remember to not use boiling water for this recipe as it can cause the yerba mate to go bitter.
10. Yerba mate is a great digestive and can be had after a heavy meal. It is also quite rich in antioxidants and helps you maintain vibrant health. You can also make this recipe in advance and place it in a flask to consume throughout the day. Be careful though- caffeine is not an ideal ingredient in our alkaline journey. Let's keep it as a treat, OK?
11. During hot days, Argentineans like to have their yerba mate (*hierba mate* in Spanish) with some apple juice. I like to add some lemon and grapefruit juice and ice cubes. Try it!

Recipe #8 Cucumber Infused Lemon Ice Tea

This is a great, natural, alkaline recipe to help you rejuvenate and replenish on a boiling hot, sunny day.

When served at a party as a soft drink, it always attracts people's attention.

One thing for sure, it can turn plain, boring water into a very interesting experience.

Serves: 2-3

Ingredients:

- 1 cup cucumber, sliced
- 4 cups filtered water
- 1 grapefruit, juiced
- 2 teaspoons of fennel seeds (or 2 teabags of fennel tea)
- stevia or maple syrup to sweeten (optional)
- ice cubes
- mint leaves, washed

Instructions:

1. Boil the water and make the fennel tea (using a teapot or a cup).
2. Set aside to cool down.
3. In the meantime, place cucumber slices and mint leaves in a jar and pour over the water.
4. Add the grapefruit juice and stevia/ or maple syrup.
5. Stir well.
6. Now, combine the infused water with fennel tea.
7. Cover the jar. Place in the fridge to make sure it cools down for approx. 1 hour.
8. Add the ice cubes, serve and enjoy!

Recipe #9 Revolutionary Rooibos Chili Tea

Rooibos is one of my favorite alkaline teas. I got really hooked on it during my visit to South Africa. It offers an amazing combination of nourishing minerals like iron, magnesium, and calcium alongside with a sweetish, delicious taste.

This recipe was created as one of my experiments, and to my surprise, the result was amazing.

I would really recommend this recipe to help you enjoy more energy and warm up on a cold, winter day. It's also great to fight off colds and flu.

Serves: 3-4

Ingredients:

- 2 tablespoons rooibos tea
- 1 tablespoon red chili flakes
- 2 cups filtered water, boiling
- 1/2 cup filtered water
- 1 lemon, juiced
- a few mint leaves to garnish

Instructions:

1. Using a teapot or a cup, combine the boiling water, rooibos tea, and chili flakes.
2. Cover and set aside for about 15 minutes.
3. Now, strain the tea and combine it with 1/2 cup filtered water and lemon juice.
4. Garnish with a few mint leaves, serve and enjoy!

Recipe #10 Horsetail Beauty Tea

This is an amazing recipe to help you detoxify your body, lose weight, reduce inflammation and get rid of water retention and cellulite. In other words, this tea can help you feel lighter and more energized.

Since it's so abundant in alkaline minerals, it can also help you grow beautiful, strong hair.

I mean...it's called Beauty Tea for a reason! Treat yourself to one cup of this amazing alkaline tea a day and you will be amazed by the results.

Serves: 2

Ingredients:

•2 tablespoons horsetail tea

•2 tablespoons mint leaves, washed

•2 tablespoons parsley leaves, washed

•2 cups filtered water, boiling

•1 inch ginger, chopped into smaller pieces

Instructions:

1. Using a teacup or a teapot, combine the horsetail, ginger, and parsley with boiling water.
2. Set aside for 10- 15 minutes.
3. Strain the tea, add in a few mint leaves and serve!
4. In case you need to, add some stevia to sweeten (although you can do very well without it).

Extra Suggestion:

Horsetail blends very well with fennel and enhances its properties. So you can also enjoy an infusion that combines fennel and horsetail tea. If your goal is natural weight loss, fat burn, more energy, healthy glowing skin, and shiny hair- then you have just found your recipe!

Enjoy!

Recipe #11 Ginger Cumin Healing Tea

This simple recipe will help you revitalize, get rid of headaches and fight off colds and flu.

Serves: 1-2

Ingredients:

- 2 inches ginger, chopped
- 2 tablespoons cumin seeds
- 2 cups filtered water, boiling
- 2 tablespoons black pepper seeds
- almond or coconut milk to taste

Instructions:

1. In a teapot, combine boiling water, ginger, cumin, and black pepper.
2. Cover and set aside for 15 minutes.
3. Strain the tea.
4. Add a bit of coconut milk to taste, serve and enjoy!

Recipe #12 Dandelion and Celery Tea

Dandelion tea is amazing for weight loss and also helps digestion.

It's re-energizing and revitalizing and can easily become your coffee substitute.

Serves: 1-2

Ingredients:

- 1 tablespoon dandelion tea
- 1 tablespoon cilantro, washed
- 1 tablespoon mint, washed
- 2 cups filtered water, boiling
- optional: stevia to sweeten

Instructions:

1. In a teapot or teacup, combine the dandelion tea, cilantro, and mint with boiling water.
2. Cover and set aside for 10-15 minutes to infuse properly.
3. Now, strain, serve and enjoy.
4. You can sweeten your tea with stevia if you want.

Recipe #13 Delicious Fennel Mint Iced Tea

If your goal is weight loss, more energy levels, better sleep, and improved digestion then fennel is an all-in-one solution.

My brother got me really hooked on it, and since then fennel has officially become my favorite herbal tea.

If I was to choose only one herb, it would probably be fennel!

Oh and rooibos...you already know I love it too. Well, both are awesome and have a sweetish taste. What more can you need?

Serves: 1-2

Ingredients:

- 1 tablespoon fennel seeds
- a handful of mint leaves, washed
- 2 cups filtered water, boiling
- ice cubes

Instructions:

1. In a teapot or a teacup, combine the boiling water with fennel seeds and mint leaves.
2. Cover and set aside for 10 minutes.
3. Then strain, and serve the tea with some ice cubes.
4. Enjoy!

Bonus recipe from Marta

Fennel essential oil recipe for your home spa.

Fennel EO is definitely one of my favorite essential oils. One of the things it's very good for is removing the sense of heaviness from your body.

Whether you suffer from water retention, swollen legs, or cellulite, or simply want to feel re-energized, I highly recommend you use fennel EO.

The best way to go about it is to make your own Fennel Energy Body Oil.

Simply combine 4 tablespoons of coconut oil, or almond oil, with 8 drops of fennel essential oil.

Massage your body after a shower or bath.

This ritual is also very relaxing and soothing for the mind. Fennel EO will also help you sleep better and reduce anxiety.

If you live in a hot climate and find yourself feeling low in energy, heavy and lethargic, then a quick cold shower and the recipe above, or its slight modification where you use aloe vera cream or gel instead of coconut or almond oil will be very helpful and alleviating.

If you are interested in learning more about EO, I highly recommend one of my previous booklets called *Essential Oils for Weight Loss*. Inside the book, I discuss the multi-functional EO in detail, while providing examples and recipes you can start applying today.

Recipe #14 Bulletproof Alkaline Cinnamon Tea

This is a simple tea that smells and tastes delicious.

Cinnamon is known for its antioxidant properties, but it is also known to regulate blood sugar levels reducing the sugar cravings that cause overeating. There is a reason why many healthy dessert recipes use cinnamon....its amazing taste makes you stop craving sugar.

This recipe takes it to a whole new level because it uses coconut oil (also great for preventing sugar cravings) and coconut milk to create a delicious, creamy consistency you are totally allowed to crave. In fact, you should. In a totally guilt-free way. Guess what tea I am going to treat myself to after finishing writing this recipe for you?

It is also associated with speeding up metabolism so is a great aid to weight loss. Oh...and it's an aphrodisiac.

Serves: 1-2

Ingredients

- 1 cup coconut milk, thin
- 1 tablespoon Ceylon cinnamon tea, or 2 cinnamon tea teabags
- 1 tablespoon coconut oil
- 1 cinnamon stick to garnish

Instructions:

1. Pour the coconut milk into a small pot and bring to the boil using medium heat.
2. When boiling, add the cinnamon tea. Stir well.
3. Reduce to low heat, cover and keep boiling on low heat for about 5 minutes.
4. Turn off the heat, add the coconut oil, and stir well.

5. Strain (if using teabags).
6. Serve in a teacup and garnish with a cinnamon stick.
7. Enjoy!

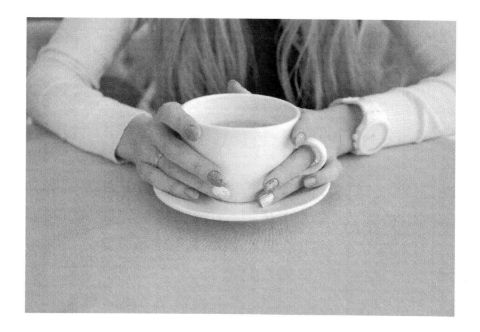

Recipe #15 Slippery Elm Digestive Wellness Infusion

Slippery elm is a tree native to North America and it has been used for various natural treatments for centuries.

It's one of the best options to help you alleviate digestive issues such as bloating. It's also great for acid reflux (in fact, it's one of the natural cures I have used to heal myself from acid reflux, alongside the healthily balanced alkaline, no coffee, and no alcohol and low-stress diet).

Aside from its main benefits, it's also helpful for a sore throat and flu.

Serves: 1-2

Ingredients

•1 tsp slippery elm bark powder (available in most wholefood shops)

•1 lemon

•1 cup of filtered, boiling water

Instructions

1.Leave the water to cool slightly.

2.Halve the lemon and squeeze 1/2 of the juice into the cooling water.

3.Slice the other 1/2 of the lemon into thick slices and add to the water.

4.Stir in the slippery elm bark powder and leave to thicken for 5-10 minutes or so.

5.Drink immediately

Recipe #16 Fenugreek and Turmeric Solution

This recipe will help you feel lighter and more energized while reducing inflammation.

It is also recommended to prevent colds and flu.

Serves: 1-2

Ingredients

- 2 cups filtered water, boiling
- 1 tbsp fenugreek seeds
- a few lime leaves, washed
- 2 slices of lime
- a 1.5-inch piece of fresh turmeric root
- 1 lemongrass stalk

Instructions

1. Bring the water to a boil using medium heat.
2. In the meantime, bash the fenugreek seeds a little, crush the lime leaves and cut the turmeric root.
3. Squash the lemongrass.
4. Add all the ingredients to boiling water. Reduce the heat to low.
5. Leave to simmer gently for 15-20 minutes so that the flavors get released.
6. Then, turn off the heat.
7. Strain all the ingredients and serve your tea in a nice teacup.
8. Garnish with some lime slices, enjoy!

Recipe #17 Lemon and Ginger All Day Energy Tonic

I absolutely love this infusion as my super hydrating morning drink. It sets my energy levels to high and is a great companion to my morning workout.

Serves: 1

Ingredients

- 1 cup filtered water
- 1-inch piece fresh ginger root
- 1-inch piece turmeric
- 10 lemon verbena leaves, washed
- 1 sliver of lemon peel
- optional- stevia or maple syrup to sweeten

Instructions

1. Boil the water using medium heat.
2. Add the ginger, turmeric, verbena leaves, and lemon peel.
3. Simmer for about 5- 10 minutes.
4. Switch off the heat and cover for about 10 minutes.
5. Strain, allow it to cool down.
6. Pour into a water jar or a glass bottle so that you always have it at hand whenever needed.

Tip from Marta: I like to make this tonic 2- 3 times a week, in larger amounts to make sure I always have some ready, especially for my morning workouts.

Recipe #18 Nettle Tea

While it will definitely hurt you to come into contact with nettle leaves in the garden, it will be very beneficial for you to enjoy their soothing, healing and alkalizing properties by using them as a tea.

Nettle tea is one of the most alkaline teas you will ever find. It's full of vitamins B and C as well as a myriad of minerals your body needs to function for you at its optimal levels.

You can also use the nettle tea infusion as a face and hair tonic. In fact, I like to use the used nettle teabags as a quick facial refresher.

You can also make nettle tea, cool it down, mix it with some lemon juice and then use it to rinse your hair after you have washed it. In fact, it's a tip and a proven recipe from my grandma.

Serves: 1-2

Ingredients

- 1 cup of filtered water, boiling
- 2 nettle teabags (you can also use the leaves, however, it's not very practical and you would need to be very careful how you handle them)
- 1 inch ginger, chopped
- slice of lemon
- optional: stevia or maple syrup to sweeten

Instructions:

1. Place the nettle teabags in a teapot or a cup with boiling water.
2. Add the ginger.
3. Cover for 10 minutes.
4. Strain, and serve with a slice of lemon.

Recipe #19 Mediterranean Alkaline Tea

This tea is an amazing combination of Mediterranean flavors. Oregano is known for its assistance with detoxifying the body with a rich helping of manganese which is an alkaline mineral.

It helps energize the body and speed up metabolism with the vitamin B it contains and boosts the immune system while helping you stay energized.

Serves: 1-2

Ingredients

- 1 cup filtered water, boiling
- 10 leaves fresh oregano, washed (or 2 tsp dried oregano)
- 3 stems of lemon thyme (or normal thyme)
- a handful of chives, washed and chopped
- 5 mint leaves (or 1 tsp dried mint)
- 2 garlic cloves, peeled

Instructions:

1. Wash all the herbs first.
2. Place in a cup or teapot and pour in the boiling water.
3. Cover and let infuse for 10-15 minutes.
4. Strain.
5. Serve warm and enjoy!

Recipe #20 Artichoke Antioxidant Tea

Artichokes are amongst the top 10 highest anti-oxidant rich foods.

Whenever I'm in need of a quick detox meal, I have a few boiled artichokes with lemon juice. There are also lots of artichoke supplements available, for example, powders and capsules.

However, my favorite way to have it is this recipe. Delicious, with energizing aroma of verbena.

Serves: 1-2

Ingredients

•2 tbsp dried or fresh artichoke leaves, washed
•8-10 leaves of lemon verbena, washed
•1 cup of filtered water

Instructions

1. Place the dried artichoke leaves and lemon verbena leaves in a teapot or cup and pour some boiling water over them.
2. Leave covered for 10 minutes.
3. Strain and enjoy!

Recipe #21 Cardamom and Vanilla Tea

Cardamom is a great, natural way to clear up coughs and flu symptoms.

It also boosts the metabolism and helps the body burn more fat, so it's definitely worth trying if you have a weight loss goal.

Ingredients

•1 tsp cardamom pods
•1 tsp vanilla extract or ½ vanilla pod
•1 cup of almond milk, unsweetened
•pinch of cinnamon

Instructions

1. Bring the almond milk to a boil, using medium heat.
2. In the meantime, crush the cardamom pods and add to the boiling milk.
3. Then, stir in the vanilla extract or if using the pod, cut the ½ vanilla pod in 1/2 and add to the milk.
4. Leave to infuse in the milk for about 15 minutes.
5. Now strain and serve with some cinnamon powder sprinkled on top.
6. Enjoy!

Recipe #22 Herbal Digestive Tea

This tea works as a natural digestive aid and it can relieve bloating and stomach cramps.

It's also great for pre-menstrual syndrome and menstrual cramps. It can also work as a relaxant, easing tension and nervous headaches.

Serves: 1-2

Ingredients

- 8 mint leaves, washed
- 2 fennel teabags (or 2 tablespoons fennel seeds)
- 1-2 dill fronds
- a handful of parsley, washed
- 2 cups of filtered water, boiling

Instructions:

1. Place the mint, fennel, dill, and parsley in a teacup or teapot.
2. Pour over some boiling water.
3. Allow to infuse for about 10 minutes. Leave for longer if you enjoy a more intense taste.
4. Strain and serve.
5. Enjoy!

Recipe #23 Rosemary Apple Tea

This herbal infusion is a warming winter drink but is equally good in the summer if you love the flavor of this drink. Rosemary is full of unique compounds and oils that provide a number of antibacterial, antifungal and anti-inflammatory properties.

Fresh apple juice will definitely spice up the taste of your tea while waking up your senses.

Serves: 1-2

Ingredients

- 1 tablespoon rosemary tea
- optional: 1 inch ginger, chopped
- ½ cup water, filtered, boiling
- ½ cup fresh apple juice
- 2 lemon slices

Instructions

1. Place the rosemary tea and ginger in a teapot or teacup.
2. Pour over the boiling water, cover and allow to infuse for 10-15 minutes.
3. Now, strain the tea and add the apple juice.
4. Serve with lemon slices and enjoy this relaxing, warm drink.

Suggestion – in the summer, serve with ice cubes as a cold iced tea.

Enjoy!

Recipe #24 Turmeric Alkaline Blend

Turmeric is well known for its anti-inflammatory properties. When blended with other ingredients in this recipe, it offers a soothing and nourishing tonic to help your body function at its optimal levels.

Grapefruit juice is very alkalizing, as it's full of alkaline minerals and low in sugar.

Serves: 1-2

Ingredients

- 1 tablespoon ginger, finely chopped
- 1 tablespoon turmeric, finely chopped
- 2 slices of lemon
- ½ cup water, filtered, boiling
- ½ cup fresh grapefruit juice (1- 2 grapefruits)
- optional: stevia or maple syrup to sweeten

Instructions:

1. Place the ginger and turmeric in a teapot or teacup and pour over some boiling water.
2. Cover and allow to infuse for about 15 minutes.
3. In the meantime, make some fresh grapefruit juice. If you don't have a juicer (I use Omega Juicer), you can easily use a simple lemon squeezer.
4. Now, strain the tea and add in the fresh grapefruit juice.
5. Stir well and if needed, sweeten with stevia or maple syrup. (To be honest, I never sweeten my tea. I am so used to its original taste.)
6. Serve with lemon slices, enjoy!

Recipe #25 Easy Sleepy Turmeric Latte

This is almost guaranteed to produce a warm, relaxed mind for a good night's sleep.

If you are craving something creamy after your dinner, you have just found your recipe!

Serves: 1-2

Ingredients

- 1 cup cashew milk
- 1 teaspoon cinnamon powder
- 1 teaspoon turmeric powder
- 1 teaspoon ginger powder
- 1 teaspoon coconut oil

Instructions:

1. Place the milk in a pot and put to boil using medium heat.
2. Add cinnamon, turmeric, and ginger.
3. Stir well, cover and leave to simmer on low heat for about 10 minutes.
4. Pour into a cup and stir in a teaspoon of coconut oil.
5. Serve warm and enjoy!

Recipe #26 Tranquility Tea

Another recipe to add to your "relax and sleep well" tea collection.

This herbal tea promotes peace and calm while seducing you with its lovely aromatic zing from the lemongrass.

You could add a pinch of stevia or maple syrup if you want to sweeten it up a little, although the chamomile does have a little sweetness anyway. You can do very well without it, or you can also serve it with some oat milk (warm oat milk helps induce sleep).

Serves: 2

Ingredients

- 1 cup of water, filtered, boiling
- 1 lemongrass stalk
- 2 tablespoons chamomile tea
- ½ cup warm oat milk (optional)
- stevia/ maple syrup (optional)

Instructions:

1. Using a teapot or a cup combine the lemongrass, chamomile and the boiling water.
2. Cover and allow to infuse for about 10 minutes.
3. Strain, and if needed add in some oat milk.
4. Stir well, serve and enjoy.
5. Sweet dreams!

Recipe #27 Blackcurrant Mint Tea Miracle

While everyone has heard of mint and mint tea, very few people have heard of blackcurrant tea.

However, in this recipe, blackcurrant plays a major role. This miraculous, caffeine-free tea is great not only for digestion but also circulation and overall wellbeing.

Enjoy!

Serves: 1-2

Ingredients

- 1 cup of water, filtered and boiling
- 2 tablespoons blackcurrant leaves (or 2 blackcurrant teabags)
- a few mint leaves

Instructions:

1. In a teapot or teacup, place the blackcurrant leaves and pour over the boiling water.
2. Cover and set aside for 10 minutes to let it infuse properly.
3. Strain the tea.
4. Serve with a few mint leaves and enjoy!

Recipe#28 Vanilla, Apricot and Mint Tea

Vanilla is a favorite flavor for many people and it's full of some wonderful health benefits.

Able to reduce inflammation and cholesterol, vanilla is perfect to enhance your wellbeing, bringing its comforting sweetness. It's also known for its antioxidant abilities so it's good for assisting your body with clearing up free radicals.

Serves: 1-2

Ingredients

- 1 cup of water, filtered, boiling
- ½ vanilla pod
- 1 apricot
- 8 mint leaves, washed

Instructions

1. Cut the vanilla pod, keeping the seeds inside*. Add to the pot or tea ball.
2. Wash, cut and remove the stone from the apricot. Cut into quarters and add to the teapot or ball.
3. Pour over the boiling water and leave to steep for 5-10 minutes
4. Serve with fresh mint leaves.

Recipe #29 Turmeric Orange Power Tea

"Wow. Wow, wow, wow! Marta, what is it? The color is just so amazing!"

That was feedback I got from a friend of mine (who at first was a bit skeptical about alkaline teas) who tried this recipe and as a consequence got hooked on alkaline drinks and recipes.

One thing is for sure - this invigorating tea will provide you with some good refreshment. Something for the senses and something for the eye- not your typical boring tea.

Turmeric acts as a great anti-oxidant and the vitamin C from the oranges also adds to the immune system boost while at the same time making this tea taste amazing.

Serves: 1-2

Ingredients

- 1 cup water, filtered
- 2 inches of fresh root of turmeric, finely chopped
- 1-2 inch ginger
- juice of 2 big oranges
- 2 lemon slices

Instructions

1. Boil the water in a pan.
2. Add the turmeric and the ginger.
3. Cover.
4. Simmer for about 20 minutes.
5. Take off the heat and allow to cool down for about 10- 20 minutes. Strain and add some fresh orange juice.
6. Serve slightly warm (but not hot), or if you're making this recipe in the summer, add some ice cubes. Enjoy!

Recipe #30 Fennel Lime Energizer a la Mojito

This recipe offers another unique combination of alkaline herbs and fruits, all in one drink.

It's an amazing combination because fennel offers a nice sweet, herbal taste and digestive properties while lime spices it up with an energizing flavor and a huge dose of vitamin C.

I am used to having this drink like it is, that is- no sweeteners at all. However, if you need to, feel free to sweeten it with some stevia. Another option is to add some crushed brown sugar (not very alkaline, but hey, every now and then it's OK, especially when you have guests).

Limes can easily be juiced through a simple lemon juicer. In case you are using Omega Juicer or a similar juicer with higher potential, you can take this drink one step further by juicing the lime with some mint leaves and 1-2 inches of ginger.

However, the basic recipe below is also great and probably easier and much more practical for most people.

Serves: 2

Ingredients

- 1/2 cup water, filtered, boiling
- 1 tablespoon fennel seeds or 2 fennel teabags
- 3 limes, juiced
- optional: stevia to sweeten
- a small handful of mint leaves

Instructions:

1. Place the fennel seeds in a teapot or teacup and pour over the boiling wter.
2. Cover and allow to infuse for 10- 15 minutes.
3. Now strain and add some mint leaves (and if needed some stevia or sugar).
4. Add the fresh lime juice.
5. Serve and enjoy!

Recipe #31 Sage Mood Enhancer

Sage is traditionally known as an uplifting herb. It can help deal with the premenstrual syndrome as well as menopause.

It blends really well with chives and ginger (both are great for anti-inflammatory properties and can also help you reduce bloating).

As an optional variation, especially for the summer, you can serve this tea with alkaline ice cubes. What are alkaline ice cubes? Simple-it's alkaline juice frozen up into ice cubes.

One of the best suggestions I could give you, especially if you have an Omega Juicer or a similar juicer that allows you to juice pretty much everything you put through it: juice large portions of lemons, ginger, turmeric, limes, and grapefruits.

Then, freeze into ice cubes that you can serve with your tea, water, and other drinks.

If you are serving guests, they will surely be surprised.

Serves: 1-2

Ingredients

- 1 cup water, filtered
- 8 sage leaves, washed and torn up (you can also use 1-2 sage teabags).
- 2-inch ginger
- 2 reeds of chives, washed and chopped into 2 cm pieces.
- optional- stevia or maple syrup to sweeten

Instructions

1. Boil the water.
2. Wash and tear up the sage leaves.
3. Wash the chives and chop into 2 cm pieces.

4. Add the herbs to a strainer or ball. You can also place them in a pot directly and strain later.
5. Pour over the water and leave to steep for 10 minutes.
6. If needed, strain.
7. Serve and enjoy!

Recipe #32 Hibiscus Floral Energizer

Hibiscus is a lovely floral, aromatic petal that is an amazing natural treatment to help you recover from a sore throat or sore gums. Not only that, but it also stimulates metabolism and is recommended for natural weight loss treatment.

And the color? Amazing! Especially if you follow my recommendation and serve it with some pomegranate juice. Absolutely miraculous combination.

Serves: 1-2

Ingredients

- 1 teaspoon dried hibiscus leaves
- pinch of stevia (optional)
- pinch of dried rose petals to garnish
- 1/2 cup filtered water, boiling
- 1/2 cup fresh, organic pomegranate juice

Instructions:

1. Place the hibiscus leaves in a teapot or cup.
2. Pour over some boiling water and cover for 10-15 minutes.
3. Strain and add in some pomegranate juice (make sure the tea is not super hot, but warm).
4. Garnish with a pinch of dried rose petals.
5. Serve and enjoy!

Optional: If needed, sweeten with stevia and add some ice cubes.

Recipe #33 Minty Melissa Relaxation Tea

This recipe combines the relaxing properties of Melissa with the soothing and healing properties of mint. A great combo to help you feel more relaxed, sleep better and soothe your digestive system too.

Serves: 1-2

Ingredients

- 1 cup of water, filtered, boiling
- 1 teabag mint tea
- 1 teabag Melissa tea
- optional: coconut or oat milk

Instructions:

1. In a teacup or pot, combine the boiling water and the mint as well as Melissa tea.
2. Cover for about 10-15 minutes.
3. Strain and mix with some oat or coconut milk (preferably warm).
4. Serve and enjoy the smoothness!

Recipe #34 Raspberry and Mint Infusion

In case you find the plain mint too boring, this recipe will spice it up. Raspberries blend really well with mint.

The color of this drink comes out really amazing and so does the flavor.

Use this recipe to soothe your digestive system while rejuvenating your mind and body.

Serves: 1-2

Ingredients

•1 cup water, filtered and boiling

•a handful of raspberries (can be frozen or fresh)

•a handful of fresh mint leaves

Instructions

1. Place the mint and raspberries in a teapot or a big teacup.
2. Pour over the water and leave to steep for 15 minutes.
3. Strain and enjoy!
4. This can be enjoyed just warm or cold with lots of ice.
5. Eat the strained raspberries as you drink your tea for optimal health benefits!

Recipe #35 Poppy Nervous Tonic

This tea is made from poppy seeds is an age-old remedy for anxiety and stress. Its healing benefits are optimized by verbena leaves and a bit of lemon to wake up the senses and help you feel uplifted to act in an empowered way.

Serves: 1-2

Ingredients

•1 tablespoon poppy seeds

•8 lemon verbena leaves

•1 cup of water, filtered, boiling

•2 slices of lemon to serve

Instructions:

1. In a teacup or teapot, combine the poppy seeds, verbena leaves, and boiling water.
2. Cover and leave to infuse for about 10 minutes.
3. Strain and serve with 2 slices of lemon.
4. If needed, sweeten a bit with stevia or maple syrup.
5. Enjoy the calmness!

Recipe #36 Tarragon Mineral Brew

Tarragon is a highly alkalizing and anti-oxidant tea due to its high mineral and vitamin content. Rich in magnesium, iron, zinc, calcium and vitamins, A, C and B-6, it will revitalize and re-energize you from the inside out, especially when you combine it with a healthy clean food diet. A word of caution though... tarragon has a very strong flavor so test this drink before allowing it to steep for too long.

Serves: 1-2

Ingredients

• 1 cup water, filtered, boiling

• 8 tarragon leaves, washed

• 6 lemon verbena leaves, washed

Instructions

1. Roughly tear the herbs and add to a cup or tea ball.
2. Pour over some boiling water.
3. Leave to steep for 5 minutes (due to the taste warning I have already mentioned, however, next time you make it feel free to experiment to see what works for you).
4. Enjoy hot and if needed sweeten with stevia, fresh apple juice or maple syrup.

Recipe #37 Spicy Anti-Oxidant Blend

I am a big fan of spices, herbs, and delicious plant-based curry recipes. The secret behind all those recipes is cumin and coriander and these can also be used to make an amazing tea recipe.

Cumin supports the digestive system while boosting immunity and acting as a great anti-oxidant, helping to mop up those free radical cells in our bodies. Coriander adds an amazing aroma and is also known for its weight loss benefits.

Serves: 1-2

Ingredients

- 2 tsp cumin seeds

- 2 tsp coriander seeds

- 1 cup of water, filtered and boiling

Instructions

1. Using a pestle and mortar, bash both types of seed up quite well to start releasing their flavor and aroma.
2. Add the seeds to a teapot or teacup with a strainer.
3. Add the boiling water to the pot and steep for 15 minutes.
4. Drink hot.
5. Enjoy!

Recipe #38 Juniper Berry Wellness Tea

Juniper berries help reduce indigestion and bloating after eating so this tea may be a good recipe to try after holiday dinners and family occasions or any not-so-alkaline, occasional indulgement.

Juniper berry is a natural source of vitamin C as well as a ton of alkaline minerals like iron, chromium, magnesium, phosphorus, potassium, and zinc.

It's got a strong, aromatic taste and smells a bit like Christmas trees. Some people enjoy such a taste while others like to add some apple juice to it. Try it to see what you prefer.

Serves: 1-2

Ingredients

- 1 cup of water, filtered, boiling
- 2 tsp juniper berries
- 2 slivers of lemon peel
- optional – stevia to sweeten

Instructions:

1. Place the juniper berries and lemon peel in a teapot or a teacup.
2. Add the water and leave covered to infuse.
3. Strain, and if needed sweeten with stevia, maple syrup or some fresh apple juice.
4. Enjoy!

Recipe #39 Ginseng Power Ginger Tea

Ginseng is one of the most popular herbal remedies to help you have more energy, revitalize your body and mind and recover after a long period of physical and mental work.

However, if you find yourself feeling anxious, ginseng may aggravate that feeling. It's also not recommended to drink ginseng tea if you are already drinking caffeine as you may find yourself overstimulated. As with any stimulant, even natural, this recipe should be avoided if you are pregnant or lactating. If you're in any doubt make sure you talk to your doctor first.

Still, most people who follow a balanced diet and don't suffer from severe anxiety or nervousness will benefit from a nice, energizing cup of ginseng tea. It could certainly be your next coffee substitute.

Serves: 1-2

Ingredients

- 1 tsp ground ginseng or 2 small roots
- 1-inch piece of fresh ginger root
- 1-inch piece of turmeric
- 1 cup of water, filtered, boiling
- 1 lemon slice
- stevia to taste

Instructions

1. Place the ginseng, ginger, and turmeric in a teapot or teacup.
2. Pour over some water.
3. Leave to infuse (covered) for about 10- 15 minutes.
4. Strain.
5. Check for sweetness and if needed sweeten with stevia.
6. Serve with a slice of lemon, enjoy!

Recipe #40 Vanilla, Orange and Sage Power

Sage is a wonderful help for a sore throat. At the same time, this tea will add some comfort to any soreness and vitamin C from the orange will help boost the immune system.

The vanilla is an amazing anti-bacterial agent and will certainly help you feel fit and energized as you deserve.

Remember, whenever you are feeling sick, it's a sign you need to take even more care of your hydration in a truly nutrient-rich and alkaline way. You need to get your body what it needs so that it can recover for you faster. Start by taking meaningful action and hydrate your mind and body.

Serves: 1-2

Ingredients

•1 cup of water, filtered, boiling
•½ vanilla pod
•8 sage leaves, washed
•1 orange or grapefruit, halved and sliced

Instructions

1. Cut the vanilla pod, leaving the seeds intact.
2. Place in a teacup or teapot and add sage.
3. Pour on the water.
4. Cover and let infuse for 15 minutes.
5. Strain and add the orange slices.
6. Serve and enjoy. Eat the orange slices as you drink the tea.

Recipe #41 Elderberry Cinnamon Dream

Elderberry has a long-standing history of being useful for coughs and colds. It's also an amazing antioxidant rich in vitamin C.

The elderberry tea has an amazing sweet taste that can be optimized and enhanced with cinnamon.

Cinnamon helps stimulate digestion and as you have already learned in one of the previous recipes in this book, it also helps prevent sugar cravings.

Drink to your health, hydrate and enjoy!

Serves: 1-2

Ingredients

- 1 cup of water, filtered, boiling
- 1 cup coconut milk, warm
- 1 handful of elderflower blossom
- ½ tsp Ceylon cinnamon
- 2 cinnamon sticks to garnish
- stevia to taste

Instructions

1. Add the elderflower blossoms to a pot or teacup.
2. Add the water and stir in the cinnamon.
3. Leave covered for 5-10 minutes until the flavors have developed.
4. Strain and add some coconut milk.
5. Serve in a teacup with a cinnamon stick inside.
6. If needed, sweeten with stevia.
7. Enjoy!

Recipe #42 Kukicha Bulletproof Anti-Inflammatory Tea

Kukicha tea is almost caffeine free (the amount of caffeine it contains is really minimal) and is jam-packed with alkaline minerals such as iron, magnesium, and calcium. This recipe is truly one of my favorite ones and can really help you quit or eliminate coffee.

Coconut oil is not to be feared at all. It's a good fat and it will help you prevent sugar cravings and energy crashes that you are prone to when you drink caffeine and sugar. (You already know this is a very short-term solution and not a very good combination to help you experience ultimate wellness and optimal energy levels.)

It's an amazing tea to enjoy on a cold winter's morning or afternoon.

It can also be turned into an iced tea. (You would simply add cold coconut milk and some ice cubes.)

Serves: 1-2

Ingredients

- 1 cup water, filtered and boiling
- 1 tablespoon kukicha tea
- 1 inch ginger, chopped
- 1 inch turmeric, chopped
- 1 teaspoon coconut oil
- quarter cup coconut milk, warm
- cinnamon stick

Instructions

1. Place the kukicha tea in a teapot or a teacup.
2. Add the ginger, turmeric, and water.
3. Cover and set aside for 15 minutes.

4. Strain, and add the coconut oil and milk.
5. Stir well.
6. Serve with a cinnamon stick, enjoy!

Recipe #43 Celery Seed and Mediterranean Broth Mineral Tea

This "tea" is almost like a broth! The basil adds a lovely fresh hit to the celery. Treat this tea as a revitalizing, plant-based broth full of minerals. You can also use it for soups and creams.

Serves: 1-2

Ingredients

- 1 cup of water, filtered, boiling
- 8 basil leaves, washed
- 1 tsp celery seeds
- 1 slice of lemon

Instructions

1. Combine the basil and celery in a teacup or teapot.
2. Pour over some boiling water, cover and leave to infuse.
3. Strain and serve with a slice of lemon, enjoy!

Recipe #44 Red Tea Creamy Dream

Red tea aka pu-erh tea is an amazing natural solution to stimulate weight loss and fat burn.

A word of caution though. Since it's not totally caffeine free it may also stimulate your nervous system. This tea is one of the "not totally caffeine free" exceptions I mentioned earlier in the intro. However, this recipe also contains fennel which is caffeine free, so the caffeine content gets drastically reduced.

Still, it's much weaker than traditional coffee. In fact, red tea is one of the teas that helped me drastically reduce my coffee intake. (I now only drink coffee occasionally.)

Personally, I love to enjoy the red tea while writing. It's one of my favorite treats and I am enjoying a cup right now.

Serves: 1-2

Ingredients:

- 1/2 teaspoon red tea
- 1 teaspoon fennel seeds
- 1 cup water, filtered and boiling
- ¼ cup coconut milk, warm
- 1 cinnamon stick to serve

Instructions:

1. Combine the fennel and red tea seeds in a teacup or teapot.
2. Pour over some boiling water and cover to infuse for 10-15 minutes.
3. Strain and add in some coconut milk for a creamy consistency.
4. Serve with cinnamon sticks.
5. Enjoy!

Recipe #45 White Tea Fat Burn Tonic

White tea is another tea that is low in caffeine and can be used to kick a coffee addiction gradually. Also, this recipe combines it with a caffeine-free herb so that the caffeine level is very, very low.

White tea is a great antioxidant and so is the ancient Mediterranean herb- marjoram. At the same time, marjoram helps reduce stress and anxiety.

Serves: 1-2

Ingredients

- 1 cup of water, filtered, boiling
- 1 teaspoon white tea
- 10 fresh marjoram leaves, washed
- stevia to sweeten (optional)

Instructions

1. Combine the white tea and marjoram in a teapot or teacup.
2. Pour over the boiling water and cover.
3. Set aside for 10- 15 minutes.
4. Strain and serve.
5. Sweeten with some stevia if needed.

Bonus Chapter: Infused Waters

This bonus chapter will inspire you to create original, fruit and herb-infused waters to help you stay hydrated.

Fruit infused waters look very attractive and always get attention at parties.

The best part?

They are very easy to prepare, will help you stay energized and get off unhealthy soft drinks and soda.

All you need is a water pitcher or a jar. You can also infuse your waters using a large glass.

Enjoy!

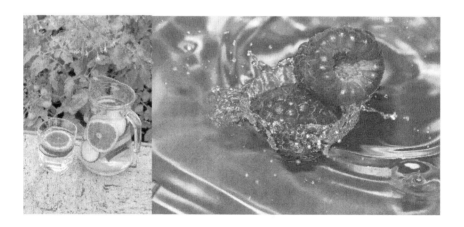

Recipe #46 Mint, Cucumber, and Lime Vitality

Refreshment is very easy with this optimal recipe.

Mint and cucumber have amazing anti-oxidant properties and it's something you can actually sense and feel while enjoying this recipe.

The lime adds a touch of sourness that works so well.

Serves: 2-4

Ingredients

- 1 handful of mint leaves, washed
- 1 cucumber, finely sliced
- 2 limes, sliced
- 4 cups water, filtered (1 liter)

Instructions

1. Place water in a suitable jug/container.
2. Add the rest of the ingredients.
3. Cover and place in a fridge for approx. 1 hour.
4. Serve and enjoy.

Serving recommendation- to enjoy the best taste, make sure you consume this recipe within 24 hours.

Recipe #47 Grapefruit Rosemary Energy

Grapefruit is a highly alkalizing citrus fruit that will help combat bloating.

At the same time, it infuses your water with vitamin C to help you boost your immune system. It blends very well with rosemary, resulting in a very original taste that will stimulate your senses.

Serves: 2-4

Ingredients

•3 sprigs of rosemary, washed
•2 grapefruits, halved and cut in small slices
•4 cups of water (1 liter), filtered

Instructions

1. Pour the water into a suitable container or jug.
2. Add the grapefruit.
3. Using a mortar, squeeze the grapefruit a bit, so that it releases more of its miraculous juices into the water.
4. Add the rosemary.
5. Cover and place in a fridge for about 1-2 hours.
6. Serve and enjoy!

Recipe #48 Raspberry and Melon Miracle Water

Either fresh or frozen raspberries could be used for the recipe. The melon adds sweetness to the raspberries and balances the flavor well. The kiwi comes in with a massive portion of vitamin C and even more flavor! The color is amazing too!

Serves: 1-2

Ingredients

- 2 handfuls of raspberries (frozen or fresh), washed
- 1/4 melon, chopped into smaller pieces
- 2 kiwis, peeled and sliced
- 4 cups water (1 liter), filtered

Instructions

1. Pour the water into a suitable container or jug.
2. Add the raspberries and, using a mortar, squash them so that they start releasing more flavor and juices into the water.
3. Now do the same with kiwis and then add the melon.
4. Cover the jar and place in a fridge for about 1- 2 hours.
5. Enjoy!

Recipe #49 Optimal Immune Booster

This is a refreshing, vitamin C packed infused water that offers ultimate hydration and replenishment. Ginger spices up the water and mango sweetens it up a bit. Perfect combo!

Serves: 1-2

Ingredients

- 1 orange, washed, peeled and sliced
- 1 lemon, washed, peeled and sliced
- ½ mango washed and sliced
- 2 inches ginger, chopped
- 4 cups water, filtered (1 liter)

Instructions

1. Pour the water into a container or jug.
2. Add all the ingredients and squash them a bit using a mortar so that they release their flavors faster.
3. Cover and place in a fridge for about 1- 2 hours.
4. Enjoy!

Bonus Chapter 2: Green Alkaline Smoothies

This bonus chapter will inspire you to try some of my best alkaline green smoothie recipes that not only hydrate and nourish you but also keep you full. In fact, many of these recipes can be used as a quick meal replacement.

It's a no-brainer, especially on a busy day, where you can give yourself the luxury of creating a healthy, alkaline and body-mind rejuvenating meal in about 5 minutes. All you need is a blender and an intention to give your body what it needs to thrive and feel amazing!

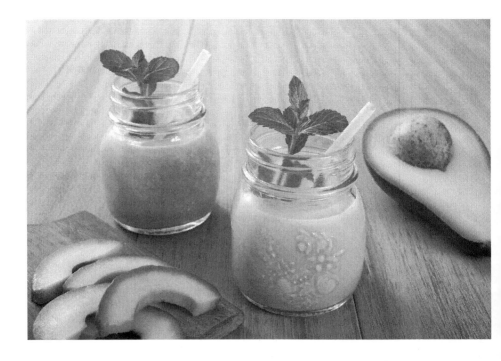

Recipe #50 Creamy Green Protein Treat

This recipe is packed with natural protein and good fats.

Not only that, but it uses spirulina which is jam-packed with micronutrients.

It's a very simple recipe with an interesting, creamy taste. Perfect for cashew addicts!

It makes a great snack and will give you a quick energy boost for sure.

Serves: 1-2

Ingredients:

- 1 cup coconut milk
- ¼ cup cashews, raw
- 1/2 teaspoon cinnamon
- 1/2 teaspoon spirulina powder

Instructions:

1. First blend the coconut milk and cashews. I like to use a Vitamix blender.
2. Now, add the cinnamon and spirulina and blend again.
3. Serve and enjoy!

Recipe #51 Vitamin C Hormone Rebalancer

This green smoothie recipe, aside from greens and fruit, is packed with vitamin C. It uses my favorite supplements-maca and ashwagandha.

Another miraculous ingredient worth mentioning is chia seed powder which is like a natural protein powder.

This is a superfood smoothie and can be a meal replacing smoothie for sure.

Serves: 1-2

Ingredients:

- 1 kiwi
- 1 ½ cups coconut milk or any other plant-based milk
- handful of spinach
- 1 green apple
- 1/2 teaspoon maca powder
- 1/2 teaspoon ashwagandha powder
- 2 teaspoons chia seeds powder

Instructions:

1. Place all the ingredients (aside from the supplements and chia seeds) in a blender.
2. Blend and then add the powders and blend again.
3. Serve and enjoy!

Recipe #52 Spicy Mediterranean Smoothie

Who said that smoothies must be sweet? Personally, I also like veggie smoothies. The trick is to make them super-tasty. That is why spices and herbs are very helpful for us. You already know that these are full of amazing detoxing and alkalizing properties.

This smoothie can also be a meal replacement and you can serve it as a nice, raw soup. Perfect for a hot summer!

Serves: 1-2

Ingredients:

- 1 ½ cups almond or coconut milk
- 1 cucumber
- 1 garlic clove, peeled
- small handful of kale
- 1/2 avocado
- 1 teaspoon chia seed powder
- handful of green olives, pitted
- another handful of green olives to garnish
- handful of almonds
- Himalayan salt to taste
- black pepper
- pinch of chili powder
- 1 teaspoon of Mediterranean herb mix (oregano and thyme are the best for this recipe).
- olive oil (approx. 1 tablespoon)

Instructions:

1. Blend the milk, cucumber, garlic, kale, avocado, and green olives.

2. Now add the chia seed powder, Himalayan salt, black pepper, and chili powder.
3. Blend again.
4. Pour in a smoothie glass or a soup plate.
5. Add in the rest of olives and almonds.
6. Stir well. Now sprinkle some Mediterranean herbs on top, add some olive oil and enjoy!

Recipe #53 Alkaline Ketogenic Super Green Smoothie

This smoothie combines the best of alkaline greens and good fats which makes it a healthy, balanced, alkaline-keto smoothie that will help you stay energized throughout the day.

Another benefit is that due to the high content of good fats it will help you reduce sugar cravings.

Serves: 1-2

Ingredients:

- 1 cup coconut milk or cashew milk
- 1 big avocado, peeled and pitted
- a few slices of tomato
- Himalayan salt
- 1 tablespoon coconut oil

Instructions:

Blend, stir well and enjoy!

Recipe #54 Alkaline Protein Massive Green Smoothie

This bonus recipe is another quick green smoothie that not only is highly alkalizing but can also be used as a meal replacement.

Enjoy!

Serves: 1-2

Ingredients:

- 1 cup almond milk
- 1 green bell pepper
- 1 cucumber
- 1/2 avocado
- 1 tablespoon chia seeds or chia seed powder
- pinch of black pepper and Himalayan salt
- 1/2 teaspoon maca powder
- 2 basil leaves to garnish

Instructions:

1. Blend the avocado, bell pepper, cucumber, and milk.
2. Now add in the chia seeds, black pepper and Himalayan salt as well as the maca powder.
3. Blend again, pour in a smoothie glass, garnish with some basil leaves and enjoy!

Conclusion

Thank you once again for taking an interest in my book.

I am really grateful for you, and I hope you were able to pick at least a few recipes you will enjoy.

My mission is to empower and inspire you to live a healthy lifestyle so that you can become the best version of yourself while enjoying the process of your transformation.

Let's finish the book with a motivational kick.

Think of all the health benefits you are creating for yourself by choosing alkaline teas and optimal hydration:

The Benefits of Alkaline Teas and Hydration:

•By adding natural drinks to your lifestyle, you will be able to stimulate natural weight loss and reduce unhealthy sugar cravings. You see, when you take care of your hydration, especially with alkaline teas and natural drinks, your body is also getting a myriad of nutrients and so it doesn't have to send you those "feed me I am so hungry" signals all the time.

•You will feel more energized for sure as your body is able to flush out toxins more quickly. Think how all areas of your life can change if you have more energy!

•Your mental and emotional health will improve with a well-hydrated body, allowing you to think better and perform better.

•You will get a ton of extra vitamins and minerals.

•Your skin will be clearer and feel smoother.

•Your cardiovascular health will be optimized.

+ You will feel stronger, and a totally new person.

So next time you feel tempted to drink something unhealthy, ask yourself, "Is it worth it? Or maybe I can choose a nutrient-packed alkaline tea or drink?"

It's all about making consistent progress and about those small daily decisions.

They will help you create what I like to call *empowering alkaline mini habits*. These, when compounded, will help you to transform in a way you never even thought was possible. It will be an amazing experience.

Finally, I need to ask you for a small favor. It will only take a few minutes of your time and will be very helpful for me at this stage. All I am asking you for is your honest review on Amazon. Your review, even a short one, can inspire someone else to start living a healthy lifestyle and enjoy the benefits of alkaline hydration.

Let's make a world a happy, healthy and more empowered place.

That collective transformation starts with small baby steps and micro-actions.

Thank you, thank you, thank you. I am really looking forward to reading your review.

Be sure to visit the next page and follow my instructions to be notified about my new books and start receiving valuable tips about the alkaline diet & lifestyle.

Xxx

Marta

Let's Keep in Touch + Alkaline Wellness Newsletter

The best way to stay in touch with me is via email.

Be sure to join my Alkaline Wellness email newsletter at:

www.HolisticWellnessProject.com/alkaline

When you sign up, you will receive free instant access to these bonus guides:

3 Free Bonus Guides

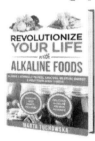 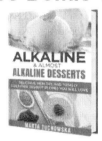 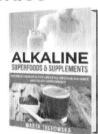

Any problems with your sign-up, please email me at:

info@holisticwellnessproject.com

Marta's Work – Holistic Wellness

To check out more of Marta's books, as well as videos, articles, programs and courses to guide you on your journey, please visit:

www.HolisticWellnessProject.com

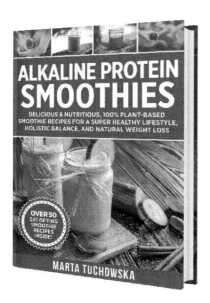 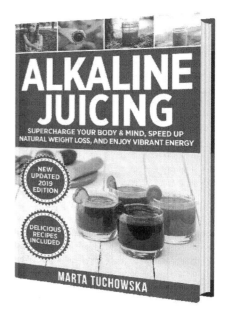

Made in the USA
Middletown, DE
18 October 2020

22149663R00061